Spanish Pocket Guide for Nurses

Donna Polverini, RN, MSN
Department of Nursing

Arthur Natella, PhD
Department of Foreign Languages

American International College
Springfield, Massachusetts

JONES AND BARTLETT PUBLISHERS
Sudbury, Massachusetts
BOSTON   TORONTO   LONDON   SINGAPORE

World Headquarters
Jones and Bartlett Publishers
40 Tall Pine Drive
Sudbury, MA 01776
978-443-5000
info@jbpub.com
www.jbpub.com

Jones and Bartlett Publishers
Canada
6339 Ormindale Way
Mississauga, Ontario L5V 1J2
Canada

Jones and Bartlett Publishers
International
Barb House, Barb Mews
London W6 7PA
United Kingdom

Production Credits
Executive Editor: Kevin Sullivan
Aquisitions Editor: Emily Ekle
Associate Editor: Amy Sibley
Production Director: Amy Rose
Editorial Assistant: Patricia Donnelly
Associate Production Editor: Amanda Clerkin
Associate Marketing Manager: Ilana Gordon
Manufacturing and Inventory Control Supervisor: Amy Bacus
Composition: NK Graphics
Cover Design: Kate Ternullo
Printing and Binding: Transcontinental
Cover Printing: Trancontinental

6048
Printed in Canada
13 12 11 10 09   10 9 8 7 6 5 4 3 2

Jones and Bartlett's books and products are available through most bookstores and online booksellers. To contact Jones and Bartlett Publishers directly, call 800-832-0034, fax 978-443-8000, or visit our website, www.jbpub.com.

Substantial discounts on bulk quantities of Jones and Bartlett's publications are available to corporations, professional associations, and other qualified organizations. For details and specific discount information, contact the special sales department at Jones and Bartlett via the above contact information or send an email to specialsales@jbpub.com.

The authors, editor, and publisher have made every effort to provide accurate information. However, they are not responsible for errors, omissions, or for any outcomes related to the use of the contents of this book and take no responsibility for the use of the products and procedures described. Treatments and side effects described in this book may not be applicable to all people; likewise, some people may require a dose or experience a side effect that is not described herein. Drugs and medical devices are discussed that may have limited availability controlled by the Food and Drug Administration (FDA) for use only in a research study or clinical trial. Research, clinical practice, and government regulations often change the accepted standard in this field. When consideration is being given to use of any drug in the clinical setting, the health care provider or reader is responsible for determining FDA status of the drug, reading the package insert, and reviewing prescribing information for the most up-to-date recommendations on dose, precautions, and contraindications, and determining the appropriate usage for the product. This is especially important in the case of drugs that are new or seldom used.

Contents

Contents

Introduction

The Latino Population

Spanish-speaking populations originate in Spain and Latin America. Although the preferred designation varies geographically, this population is most commonly referred to as "Latino" or "Hispanic."

Nurses typically encounter clients who have developed a language known as Spanglish, a combination of Spanish and English words. Spanish, like other languages, has many dialects, and words can vary from place to place. It is necessary to ensure that the nurse is being understood and understands the client. For example, in Puerto Rican culture, nonverbal behavior and symbolism are embedded in the language. Hand gestures and facial expressions are used to communicate and must be understood by the nurse, and clarification is often needed. There will be times when family may be able to assist in communication. It is not uncommon to have children present as interpreters. Age appropriateness should be considered, along with the content of the discussion. There are other times when it will be necessary to enlist the aid of an interpreter or translator.

The nurse should be clear that he/she does not speak Spanish. Ethically and legally, the nurse should enlist an interpreter or translator when necessary. (See disclaimer.) To facilitate communication, the nurse should

- Speak slowly and clearly.
- Give instructions one at a time.
- Utilize family members when appropriate for communication.
- Utilize an interpreter or translator when necessary, particularly when dealing with legal matters such as patient teaching, consent for treatment, and discharge planning.

How to Use This Book

This pocket manual was created to assist in the daily communication of the Spanish-speaking client. Each section contains the most commonly used terms and questions daily encountered in the acute care setting. It is not intended to be all-encompassing, or it would expand beyond the usefulness of a pocket manual. Each question is formatted to elicit a "yes," "no," "maybe," or "I don't know" response.

At times, terms are repeated in a particular section to avoid cross-referencing. At other times, the reader will need to refer to another section; for instance, assessments regarding pain are found in Chapter 1, "Pain." Each chapter presents cultural notes, followed by helpful hints when appropriate. Remember that although a particular culture may have general characteristics, individual variations may occur and no assumptions should be made without communicating with the client.

General Cultural Observations

Religion: The majority of Latinos are Christian and are deeply invested in their religion. At times, illness, disease, and death are considered acts of God, sometimes as punishment for wrongdoings. This may impact their ability to engage in activities to prevent illness or improve their health. The nurse should

- Respect the role of religion in the client's health.

- Refrain from removing religious artifacts without permission.
- Understand that faith often gives the client an external locus of control.

Time: Latinos often focus on present time and may not always be on time for appointments. Recurring tardiness may make it difficult for the Latino client to cooperate in wellness programs or health promotion activities. The nurse should

- Focus on short-term problems when educating the client.
- Educate the client with specifics about the detrimental effects of poor disease management.
- Stress the fact that tardiness may mean loss of appointments and meetings with physicians and other healthcare professionals.

Respect and Courtesy: Out of courtesy, many Latinos will pretend to understand when, in fact, they do not. To avoid being rude, they may hesitate to ask the nurse to slow down or to repeat what has been said. They may feel the need to "save face." Arguments and direct confrontation are considered rude. Kidding is reserved for family and friends. Latinos may tend to engage in small talk before getting to the business at hand. Many times, food is offered by family members to healthcare providers as gifts. The nurse should

- Address the client formally until a relationship is established.
- Establish familiarity before beginning assessments.
- Postpone kidding around with the client until a relationship has been established.
- Avoid confrontation.
- Accept gifts of food as a sign of respect and appreciation.

Family: Family is important in Hispanic culture. Latinos generally have a great need for togetherness and will have many extended family members arrive at the hospital in great numbers. Typically, the man is the head of the household and the decision maker, but decisions are made within the family context. Women are the caregivers and provide childcare. The eldest female is considered the expert in childcare. Nurses should

- Respect the need for family presence.

- Enlist family members to assist in the client's care, such as bathing, feeding, and ambulation, to help foster the client's trust and respect.
- Provide space within the client's room and the family waiting room for relatives and friends.
- Explain the need for hospital policies while respecting cultural family values.
- Accept the male as the financial decision maker.
- Consider the eldest female as the expert in child care.

Alternative therapies: Latinos often use alternative therapies first and then turn to Western medicine. A **partera** (midwife) or **curandero** (folk healer) may be used. Folk medicine may include the use of herbs, massage, religious artifacts, and/or chiropractors. Clients may be hesitant to admit to use, for fear that such practices will no longer be allowed. Encourage a mix of alternative therapies and Western medicine, as long as the combination, or the therapies, alone, are not contraindicated. The nurse should

- Establish a relationship with folk healers and others providing care to the client.
- Be culturally sensitive when questioning clients about herbs or alternative therapy use.
- Integrate alternative therapies with Western medicine when possible.

The Spanish Language

Phonetic pronunciation is provided with the Spanish translation, but it may be helpful to understand a few basic rules of the language:

- Vowels in Spanish are always pronounced in the same way:

    A is pronounced "ah" as in the exclamation "ah."

    E is pronounced "e" as in the word "bet."

    I is pronounced "ee" as in the word "deep."

    O is pronounced "o" as in the word "over."

    U is pronounced "oo" as in the word "tune."

- Most consonants are pronounced as they are in English with the following exceptions:

    "J" is pronounced by letting a flow of air come out of the mouth just as Santa Claus pronounces the letter "h" when he says "ho ho ho!"

Double **ll** is pronounced like a "y" in English.

The letter **h** is silent. It is not pronounced.

The letter **r** is trilled like the "r" in the word "throw."

A double **rr** is trilled at least twice as long as a single **r**.

j is pronounced like "h."

g is pronounced like the English "h" when it comes before "e" or "i." Before letters "a," "o," or "u," it has a hard "g" sound as in the word "get."

c before "e" and "i" is pronounced like the letter "s" as in the word "sent." In most of Spain, however, this letter is pronounced as "th."

c coming before "a," "o," or "u" is pronounced as a hard "c" sound, as in the word "cat."

■ Unlike English, nouns in Spanish have genders:

Nouns ending in **a** are usually feminine.

Nouns ending in letter **o** are usually masculine.

The word "the" for masculine nouns is **el** (**el libro,** "the book").

The word "the" for feminine nouns is **la** (**la casa,** "the house").

- Plurals of nouns ending in vowels are formed by adding the letter **s** to the word:

  The word for plural masculine "the" is **los** (**los libros**).

  The word for plural feminine "the" is **las** (**las casas**).

- Object pronouns: When an action refers to a thing or person, that thing or person is an object. Instead of the name of such a thing or person, words like "him," "her," or "it" (pronouns) may be used, and the word used depends on the gender of the object or person.

Singular

me	me
te	you (*familiar*)
lo	him, you (formal) or it (*masculine*)
la	her, you (formal) or it (*feminine*)

Plural

nos	us
los	them, you (*plural*) (*masculine*)
las	them, you (*plural*) (*feminine*)

When addressing both males and females together in a group, the masculine form is used. For example:

Yo te hablo.	I speak to you. (*familiar form of you*)
Él me habla.	He speaks to me.
Tengo que examinarlo.	I have to examine you. (*speaking to a male patient*)
Tengo que examinarla.	I have to examine you. (*speaking to a female patient*)

Authors' Note

This pocket guide is intended for use in daily communication with Spanish speaking patients. It may also be helpful when an interpreter is not available. It is the nurse's legal responsibility to determine when the use of a translator or interpreter is required. Examples of these circumstances will include, but are not limited to, patient teaching and discharge planning.

Chapter 1

Pain

Cultural Notes: The personal quality known as
machismo is a well-known characteristic of men
in the Spanish-speaking world. Coming from the
Spanish word for "male," **machismo** refers to an
exaggerated or self-conscious show of personal
toughness and/or aggressiveness, often
demonstrated in an apparent lack of fear or any
visible display of emotion, even in extreme
situations. This can of course relate to medical
situations when a **macho**-oriented patient may
not complain of any pain when in fact he does
feel pain, perhaps even to a great degree.

Latina women may tend to be very expressive,
loud, and moan when in pain. Crying and
moaning may be employed as a means of
relieving pain, not a way of expressing pain.

Helpful Hints:

- Assure the client that feeling pain is a normal part of medical conditions and that giving an indication of painful symptoms is neither unusual nor a sign of weakness.
- Explain that unwillingness to admit to pain may be due to cultural conditioning.
- Explain that admission of pain may be absolutely vital to proper diagnosis and that openness and honesty is needed.
- Do not assume nonverbal behavior is an admission of pain.

3 | Pain

Dolor (*Dough-lore*)

Are you in pain?	**¿Tiene Usted dolor?** *(Tee-en-eh oo-steth doh-lohr?)*
Point to the pain.	**Señáleme el dolor.** *(Sehn-yahl-eh-meh l doh-lohr.)*
Does it hurt when I touch here?	**¿Le duele cuando lo/la toco allí?** *(Leh d-weh-leh k-wan-doh loh/la toh-koh ay-ee?)*
Is the pain:	**¿Es el dolor?** *(s el doh-lohr?)*
dull?	**¿tenue?** *(teh-oo-weh)*
sharp?	**¿agudo?** *(Ah-goo-thoh)*
burning?	**¿ardiente?** *(ar-dee-ehn-teh)*
crushing?	**¿que no te deja respirar?** *(keh noh teh deh-ha res-peer-ar?)*

deep	**¿profundo?** *(proh-foon-doh.?)*
on the skin	**¿en la piel?** *(n la pee-L?)*
intermittent	**¿intermitente?** *(een-tehr-meet-ehn-teh?)*
constant	**¿constante?** *(kohn-stahn-teh.?)*
Does the pain radiate? (go somewhere else)?	**¿Va el dolor de un lugar a otro?** *(Va-l doh-lohre deh oon loo-gar aho-troh)*
Point to where the pain radiates.	**Muéstreme con el dedo el lugar donde llega el dolor.** *(Moo-ehs-tra-meh kohn L deh-doh-l loo-gar don-deh yeh-ga-l doh-lohr)*
Is the pain worse when you	**¿Se intensifica el dolor cuando Usted?** *(Seh in-ten-see-fee-ka-l doh-lohr k-wan-doh oo-steth)*
move?	**se mueve?** *(seh moo-eh-veh.?)*

Pain

Pain	Pain
breathe?	**se respira?** *(seh res-peer-ah?)*
lie down?	**se acuesta?** *(seh a-kwahes-tah?)*
Can you rate your pain?	**¿Puede Usted calificar la intensidad del dolor?** *(Poo-eh-deh oo-steth kal-ee-fee-kar la een-ten-see-dath del doh-lohr?)*
Point to the number *(Refer to number chart.)*	**Señale el número.** *(Sen-ya-leh L noom-ehr-oh.)*
No pain 0 — 5 — 10 Worst pain	**(Ningún dolor)** *(Neen-goon doh-lohr-eh-oh)* 0 — 5 — 10 **El peor dolor** *(L pay-or doh-lohr dee-ace)*
Do you need medicine for the pain?	**¿Necesita Usted medicina para el dolor?** *(Ness-eh-see-ta oo-steth med-ee-seen-ah par-ah L doh-lohr)*

Chapter 2

Respiratory

Cultural Note: Clients of Hispanic origin may exhibit signs of accelerated breathing or even hyperventilation due to emotional conditions.

Helpful Hints:

- Offer special assurances about the client's condition as much as possible.
- Allow client as much time as possible to calm the emotional state to reduce the breathing rate.

Respiratory

Respiratory	Respiratory
Are you having trouble breathing?	**¿Tiene problemas al respirar?** *(Tee-en-eh proh-bleh-mas al res-peer-ahr?)*
Do you need a breathing treatment?	**¿Necesita un tratamiento para respirar?** *(Ness-eh-see-tah un tra-ta-mee-en-toh pa-ra res-peer-ahr?)*
Does it hurt to breathe?	**¿Le duele cuando respira?** *(Leh dwell-eh kwon-doh res-peer-ah?)*
Are you coughing?	**¿Está tosiendo?** *(S-ta toh-see-en-doh?)*
A lot?	**¿Mucho?** *(Moo-choh?)*
Are you coughing up sputum?	**¿Está tosiendo con flema?** *(S-tah toh-see-en-doh fleh-ma?)*
A lot?	**¿Mucho?** *(Moo-choh?)*
Is it thick?	**¿Está gruesa?** *(S-ta groo-eh-sa?)*

Respiratory

What color is it?	**¿De qué color es?** *(Day k koh-lohr s?)*
(See Appendix B)	
I'm going to give you oxygen.	**Le voy a dar oxigeno.** *(Leh voy a dar ohk-z-hen-o.)*
I'm going to listen to your chest.	**Voy a escuchar su pecho.** *(Voy a s-koo-char soo peh-choh.)*
Take a deep breath.	**Respire fuerte.** *(Res-peer-a foo-ehr-teh.)*
Cough.	**Tosa.** *(Toh-sa.)*
Do you smoke cigarettes?	**¿Fuma Usted cigarillos?** *(Foo-ma oo-steth see-gar-ee-yos?)*
How many packs a day?	**¿Cuántas cajetillas cada día?** *(Kwan-tas ka-heh-tee-yas ka-tha dee-a?)*
How long have you been smoking?	**¿Desde cuándo fuma Usted?** *(Des-deh kwan-doh foo-ma oo-steth?)*

Chapter 3

Cardiovascular

Cultural Notes: Some of the foods that Latinos eat tend to be fried foods or foods that are high in sodium such as **"pernil"** (a salty type of meat) or **"mole,"** (a spicy sauce) among others. Strong coffee is often part of the typical diet in these populations.

It is important to watch the foods that friends and family members bring to the patient as an expression of love and concern because they may consider that hospital food is too bland. Make sure that patients are not eating foods that are prohibited by their restricted diets. There is a high incidence of hypertension and cardiovascular disease in the Latino population that is compounded by diets that are high in fats and sodium.

Helpful Hints:

- Respect cultural diet preferences while attempting to educate about harmful effects.
- Be alert to the impact of excessive intake of caffeine on the cardiac system. Monitor pulse for rate, rhythm, and quality.
- Monitor blood pressure.
- Educate the client about the short-term benefits of dietary and lifestyle changes. Be culturally sensitive and non-judgmental.

(See chapters on pain and respiratory for further assessment.)

Cardiovascular	Cardiovascular
Are you very tired?	**¿Está Usted cansado/a?** (S-ta oo-steth kan-sa-thoh/tha)
Do you feel faint?	**¿Siente Usted que va a desmayarse?** (See-en-teh oo-steth k va a des-ma-yar-seh?)
Do you have chest pain?	**¿Tiene Usted dolor en el pecho?** (Tee-en-eh oo-steth doh-lohr n l peh-cho?)
Do you feel palpitations?	**¿Tiene Usted palpitaciones?** (Tee-en-eh oo-steth pal-pee-ta-cee-oh-nehs?)
Are you short of breath?	**¿Tiene Usted problemas al respirar?** (Tee-en-eh oo-st-eth proh-blehm-a al res-peer-ahr?)
Do you have swelling in your feet?	**¿Están hinchados los pies?** (S-tan in-cha-thohs los pee-ace?)
Do you have swelling in your hands?	**¿Están hinchadas las manos?** (S-tan in-cha-thahs las-man-ohs?)
Do you have pain in your calves?	**¿Tiene Usted dolor en las pantorrillas?** (Tee-en-eh oo-steth doh-lohr n las pan-tor-ee-yas?)

Chapter 4

Gastrointestinal

Cultural Notes: Latin American cuisine is usually very high in fats and condiments. Many people of Hispanic heritage also frequently drink coffee with each meal, as well as at coffee breaks and with snacks, so that it is not unusual for many individuals to drink as many as eight or nine cups of strong black coffee in a day. Latinos also often drink herbal teas to cure stomach problems. These teas include such teas as "té de boldo" (to treat constipation and colic), "té de manzilla" (chamomile tea), and "té de cascara sagrada" (to treat constipation.) Latino families also believe that a robust, typical diet—including ingestion of strong coffee—is essential for recovery. There is also a high incidence of lactose intolerance in Mexican Americans. Those of Puerto Rican descent are known to suffer from **empacho,** a folk disease caused by lack of food digestion that leads to painful stomach cramps.

Spicy foods are part of the typical Latino diet and may cause gastric symptoms and pain.

It is possible that a male Hispanic client may be so modest as to avoid having a bowel movement on a bedpan or commode thus, the client may choose not to move his bowels at all during the entire hospitalization.

Helpful Hints:

- Emphasize the importance of following what may be a bland hospital diet.
- Be aware that often Latino families may wish to sneak in additional foods for the recovery of the client.
- Educate the client and family about any dietary restrictions.
- Evaluate for gastric disorders caused by intake of strong coffee and spicy foods.
- Assess for lactose intolerance.
- Accept gifts of food as a sign of respect and appreciation.
- Encourage male family members to assist in care of male family members.
- Assess bowel sounds appropriately.
- Enlist male family members to assist those on restricted activity.

Do you have pain in your abdomen? (See chapter 1)	**¿Tiene Usted dolor en el estómago?** (Tee-en-eh oo-steth doh-lohr n L s-toh-ma-goh)
Do you have nausea?	**¿Tiene Usted náusea?** (Tee-en-eh oo-steth now-see-a?)
Have you vomited?	**¿Ha vomitado Usted?** (A voh-mee-ta-thoh oo-steth?)
When?	**¿Cuándo?** (Kwan-doh?)
How many times?	**¿Cuántas veces?** (Kwan-tas veh-sehs?)
What color was it?	**¿De qué color era?** (Deh k koh-lohr ehr-a?)
Was there blood in it?	**¿Había sangre en el vómito?** (A-bee-a san-greh n-l vo-mee-toh?)
Do you have trouble swallowing?	**¿Tiene Usted problemas al tragar?** (Tee-en-eh oo-steth proh-blehmas al-tra-gar?)

Gastrointestinal	Gastrointestinal
Do you have pain when you swallow?	¿Siente Usted dolor al tragar? (See-en-teh oo-steth doh-lohr al tra-gar?)
Do you have indigestion?	¿Tiene Usted acedia? (Tee-en-eh oo-steth ah-seh-dee-a?)
Have you gained weight?	¿Ha ganado Usted peso? (A gan-a-though oo-steth peh-so?)
How many pounds?	¿Cuántas libras? (Kwan-tas lee-bras?)
Have you lost weight?	¿Ha perdido Usted peso? (A per-dee-thoh oo-steth peh-so?)
Do you have pain after you eat?	¿Tiene Usted dolor después de comer? (Tee-en-eh oo-steth doh-lohr des-poh-weh deh koh-mehr?)
Do you drink coffee? Tea?	¿Bebe Usted café? Té? (Beh-beh oo-steth ka-feh? Tay?)
How many cups a day?	¿Cuántas tazas al día? (Kwan-tas ta-sas al dee-ah?)

How often do you have a bowel movement?	**¿Cada cuándo tiene Usted evacuaciones?** *(Ka-tha kwan-thoh tee-n-eh oo-steth ee-vac-oo-ah-see-ohn-ehs?)*
Is there blood in it?	**¿Tiene sangre en el excremento?** *(Tee-en-eh san-greh n L x-cra-men-toh?)*
Do you have hemorrhoids?	**¿Tiene Usted hemorroides?** *(Tee-en-eh oo-steth hem-o-royth-ehs?)*

Chapter 5

Metabolic/ Endocrine

Cultural Note: There is a high incidence of diabetes among the Latino population. There is also a tendency towards obesity, which is seen as a sign of prosperity within Latino culture.

Helpful Hints:

- Be alert for signs, symptoms, and complications related to diabetes in this population.
- Be sensitive to cultural beliefs related to weight. Educate the client about the ability to manage diabetes and related complications with weight reduction and exercise.

Are you diabetic?	**¿Tiene Usted diabetes?** *(Tee-en-eh oo-steth dee-ah-beh-tehs?)*
Do you take insulin?	**¿Toma insulina?** *(Toh-ma een-soo-leen-ah?)*
Do you take pills for your diabetes?	**¿Toma pastillas para la diabetes?** *(Toh-ma pas-tee-yas pa-ra la dee-ah-beh-tehs?)*
Do you feel: hungry?	**¿Tiene hambre?** *(Tee-en-eh am-breh?)*
nervous?	**¿Está nervioso/a?** *(S-ta nehrvee-oh-soh/ah?)*
dizzy?	**¿Está mareado/a?** *(S-ta mar-eh-ath-oh/ah?)*
confused?	**¿Está confundido/a?** *(S-ta kohn-foon-dee-thoh/ah?)*
anxious?	**¿Tiene ansiedad?** *(Tee-en-eh ahn-see-ah-dath?)*

Metabolic/Endocrine	Metabolic/Endocrine
weak?	**¿Está débil?** *(S-ta deh-beel?)*
hungry?	**¿Tiene hambre?** *(Tee-en-eh am-breh?)*
thirsty?	**¿Tiene sed?** *(Tee-en-eh seth?)*
I need to test your blood sugar.	**¿Necesito chequear su azúcar.** *(Ness-eh-see-toh cheh-kehar soo a-soo-kar.)*
Do you have trouble with your thyroid?	**¿Tiene problemas con la tiroides?** *(Tee-en-eh pro-bleh-mas kon la tee-roi-thehs.)*
Do you take medication for your thyroid?	**¿Toma medicina para la tiroides?** *(To-ma mehd-eh-see-na pa-ra la tee-roi-thehs?)*

Chapter 6

Renal

Cultural Note: Both Latino men and women, may be very modest. There is high incidence of hypertension and diabetes in this population, which are both risk factors for renal disease.

Helpful Hints:

- Provide same-sex health care providers when possible.
- Enlist the assistance of same-sex family members when appropriate.
- Assess urine patterns and kidney function carefully.

Renal	Renal
Have you had problems with your kidneys?	**¿Tiene Usted problemas con los riñones?** (*Tee-en-eh oo-steth pro-blehm-as kohn lohs reen-yon-ehs?*)
Have you had problems with your bladder?	**¿Ha tenido problemas con la vejiga?** (*A ten-ee-thoh proh-blehm-as kohn la veh-hee-ga?*)
Do you have trouble controlling urination?	**¿Tiene problemas al tratar de controlar la orina?** (*Tee-en-eh proh-blehm-as al tra-tar deh kohn-trohl-ar la o-reen-na?*)
Is urination painful?	**¿Siente dolor al orinar?** (*See-en-teh doh-lohr al o-ree-nar?*)
Is urination difficult?	**¿Es difícil orinar?** (*S dee-fee-seel o-ree-nar?*)
Do you need to urinate?	**¿Necesita orinar?** (*Ness-eh-see-ta o-ree-nar?*)

Is your urine cloudy?
¿Está oscura la orina?
(S-ta oh-skoo-rah la oh-ree-na?)

Is there blood in your urine?
¿Hay sangre en la orina?
(Eye-san-greh n la o-reen-a?)

Does it burn when you urinate?
¿Siente una quemazón al orinar?
(See-en-teh oo-na k-ma-sohn al o-ree-nar?)

Does it itch when you urinate?
¿Siente una comezón al orinar?
(See-en-teh oo-na ko-meh-sohn al o-ree-nar?)

Chapter 7

Reproductive—Male

Cultural Notes: Male clients may refuse a physical exam out of modesty. Content of topic to be discussed should be considered when assessing the need for an interpreter. As a result of **machista** culture, Latino men may not be accustomed to using condoms.

Helpful Hints:

- Attempt to provide a male health care provider.
- Consider the topic to be discussed, as well as the gender of the client, when considering the need for an interpreter .
- Avoid judgmental tones when addressing the use of condoms. Explain health concerns regarding sexually transmitted diseases versus birth control.

Are you able to urinate?	**¿Puede Usted orinar?** (Poo-weh-theh oo-steth oh-reen-ar?)
Is urination painful?	**¿Siente Usted dolor al orinar?** (See-en-teh oo-steth doh-lohr al oh-reen-ar?)
Is your urine cloudy?	**¿Está oscura la orina?** (S-ta oh-skoor-ah la oh-reen-ah?)
Is there blood in your urine?	**¿Hay sangre en la orina?** (Eye san-greh n la oh-reen-ah?)
Are you able to have an erection?	**¿Puede Usted hacer una erección?** (Poo-weh-they oo-steth ah-ser oo-na ehr-ehk-see-ohn?)
Are you able to have sexual relations?	**¿Puede Usted tener relaciones sexuales?** (Poo-weh-theh oo-steth ten-eh reh-las-ee-ohn-ehs sex-oo-al-ehs?)
With a woman?	**¿Con una mujer?** (K-ohn oo-na moo-hehr?)

Reproductive —Male	Reproductive —Male
With a man?	**¿Con un hombre?** *(K-ohn oon ohm-breh?)*
With many people?	**¿Con mucha gente?** *(K-ohn moo-cha hen-teh?)*
Do you use condoms?	**¿Usa Usted condones?** *(Oo-sa oo steth cohn-dohn-ehs?)*
Do you have any sexually transmitted diseases?	**¿Tiene enfermedades que se transmiten sexualmente?** *(Tee-en-eh n-fehr-meh-dath-ehs k say trans-moot-tehn sex-oo-al-men-teh?)*

Chapter 8

Reproductive— Female

Gynecology

Cultural Notes: In some Spanish-speaking countries, the word **regla** is used for "period;" in others the word used is **menstruacion.** In Hispanic countries, "aborto" is used for both "abortion" and "miscarriage."

Women may have difficulty being examined due to modesty and should be assigned a female health care provider or a female should assist in the examination. In some Latino cultures, menstruating women may be discouraged from walking barefoot, washing their hair, or taking showers or baths, and they may have heard that sour or iced foods may cause menstrual blood to coagulate. These beliefs may not apply to younger generations of the population, but may be practiced out of respect for elders.

Topics related to sexual behavior or that carry a stigma (such as AIDS) may be difficult for the Hispanic client to discuss with a family member present. It would be more appropriate at this time to use an interpreter.

Helpful Hints:

- Attempt to provide a female health care provider, or have a female assist in the examination.

- Expose only that part of the body being examined.

- Ask the client about particular beliefs related to menstruation, and respect the client's cultural needs.

- Consider the topic to be discussed, as well as the gender of the client, when considering the need for an interpreter.

(Refer to Appendix B for time, color, numbers, vocabulary and expressions.)

Are you in menopause?	**¿Está Usted en la menopausia?** (S-ta oo-steth n la men-oh-paus-ee-a?)
Have you missed a period?	**¿No ha tenido su regla o menstruación?** (No a ten-ee-thoh soo-reg-la oh men-stroo-ah-see-ohn?)
When was your last period?	**¿Cuándo fue su última regla/menstruación?** (K-wan-doh foo-eh soo ul-tee-ma reh-gla/men-stroo-ah-see-ohn?)
Are you having a period now?	**¿Tiene la regla o está menstruando ahora?** (Tee-en-eh la reg-la o-s-ta menstroo-ahn-thoh ah-ohr-a?)
When did your period start?	**¿Cuándo empezó a reglar o cuándo empezó su menstruación?** (Kwan-doh m-peh-soh a reg-lar o kwan-doh m-peh-soh soo men-stroo-ah-see-ohn?)

Reproductive —Female	Reproductive —Female
Are you pregnant?	**¿Está embarazada?** *(S-ta m–bar-ah-sa-tha?)*
When is your baby due?	**¿Cuándo nace su bebé?** *(Kwan-doh na-seh soo-beh-beh?)*
Do you have regular periods?	**¿Tiene reglas o menstruaciones regulares?** *(Tee-en-eh reg-las o men-stroo a-see-ohn-ehs reg-oo-lar-ehs?)*
Do you bleed between your periods?	**¿Tiene sangrado entre regla y regla o menstruación?** *(Tee-en-eh san-gra-thoh en-treh reg-la eh reg-la oh men-stroo-a-see-ohn?)*
Do you have regular periods?	**¿Tiene reglas regulares o menstruaciones regulares?** *(Tee-en-eh reg-las reg-oo-lar-ehs o men-stroo-ah-see-ohn-ehs reg-oo-lar-ehs?)*

How many days do your periods last?	**¿Cuánto tiempo le dura su regla o menstruacion?** *(Kwan-toh tee-m-poh leh du-ra soo reg-la oh men-stroo-ah-see-ohn?)*
Do you have heavy bleeding with your periods?	**¿Tiene mucho sangrado durante su regla o menstruación?** *(Tee-en-eh mu-cho san-gra-thoh door-an-te-soo reg-la oh men-stroo-a-see-ohn?)*
Do you have painful periods?	**¿Tiene reglas o menstruaciones dolorosas?** *(Tee-en-eh men-stroo-a-see-ohn-ehs doh-lohr-oh-sas?)*
Do you have any vaginal sores?	**¿Tiene úlceras o verrugas en la vagina?** *(Tee-en-eh ul-ser-as oh veh-oo-gas en la va-heen-ah?)*
Do you have any sexually transmitted diseases?	**¿Tiene enfermedades que se transmiten sexualmente?** *(Tee-en-eh n-fehr-meh-dath-ehs k say trans-moot-tehn sex-oo-al-men-teh?)*

Reproductive —Female

Reproductive —Female	
Do you have unusual vaginal discharge?	**¿Tiene y flujo de la vagina?** *(Tee-en-eh floo-hoh deh la va-heen-ah?)*
Do you use tampons? Pads?	**¿Usa tampones o toallas sanitarias?** *(Oo-sa tam-pohn-ehs oh to-ah-yas san-ee-taree-as?)*
Do you have sexual intercourse?	**¿Tiene relaciones sexuales?** *(Tee-en-eh reh-las-eh-ohn-ehs sex-oo-al-ehs?)*
With a woman?	**¿Con una mujer?** *(Kown oo-na moo-hehr?)*
With a man?	**¿Con un hombre?** *(Kown oon om-breh?)*
With many people?	**¿Con mucha gente?** *(Kown moo-cha hen-teh?)*
Do you use birth control pills?	**Usa Usted pastillas anticonceptivas?** *(Oo-sa oo-steth pa-stee-yas an-tee-cohn-cep-teev-as?)*

Condones?	**¿Condones?** *(kohn-dohnehs?)*
An IUD?	**¿Un IUD?** *(Oon EE-OO-DEH?)*
A diaphragm?	**¿Un diafragma?** *(Oon dia-frag-ma?)*
How many children do you have?	**¿Cuántos hijos tiene?** *(kwan-tohs ee-hohs tee-n-eh?)*
Have you had an abortion?	**¿Ha tenido algún aborto?** *(A ten-ee-thoh al-gun ah-bohr-toh?)*
How many?	**¿Cuántos?** *(Kwan-tohs?)*
Have you had a miscarriage?	**¿Ha tenido un aborto involuntario?** *(A ten-ee-thoh oon a-bor-toh een-vol-oon-tar-ee-oh?)*
How many?	**¿Cuántos?** *(Kwan-tohs?)*
When?	**¿Cuándo?** *(Kwan-doh?)*

Obstetrics

Cultural Notes: In the Hispanic culture the astrological or numerological significance of certain birth dates may have a special importance. Family members may have a preference that a baby be born on a certain date and therefore may wish for medical personnel to attempt to rush or delay the delivery of a baby.

In Mexican American culture, there may be fear of **mal ojo** ("evil eye"), a folk illness affecting children and infants. There is a high incidence of spina bifida in Mexican Americans, especially in the state of Texas.

Latinos typically want their husbands, and possibly female relatives, present during the delivery. Latino women want reassurance, love, and affectionate talk during labor.

Helpful Hints:

- Be sensitive to the cultural concerns regarding the delivery date and educate the client about the harmful potential.
- When complimenting, looking at, or caring for the infant, touch or pat the infant to ward off evil spirits.
- Encourage family presence and support during labor and delivery.
- Be alert for the possibility of birth defects.

When is your baby due?	**¿Cuándo nace su bebé?** *(Kwan-doh na-seh soo beh-beh?)*
How far apart are the contractions?	**¿Qué tan separadas están las contracciones?** *(K tan sep-r-ath-as s-tan las kohn-track-see-ohn-ehs?)*
Did your water break? When? (*Refer to Appendix B on time.*)	**¿Ya se rompió la fuente? ¿Cuándo?** *(Ya say rohm-p-oh la foo-when-teh? Kwan-doh?)*
I need to examine you.	**Tengo que examinarla.** *(Ten-goh k x-am-een-ar-la.)*
Put your feet here.	**Póngase los pies aquí.** *(Pohn-ga-seh lohs pee-ehs a-kee.)*
Move down.	**Póngase abajo.** *(Pohn-ga-seh ah-bah-hoe.)*
You are dilated ____ centimeters.	**Ya tiene una dilatación de ____ centímetros.** *(Ya tee-en-eh oo-na dee-la-taz-ee-ohn deh ____ sen-tee-meh-trohs.)*

Reproductive—Female			Reproductive—Female	
1 **uno** (oo-noh)	2 **dos** (dohs)	3 **tres** (trehs)	4 **cuatro** (kwah-troh)	5 **cinco** (seen-koh)
6 **seis** (say-s)	7 **siete** (see-et-teh)	8 **ocho** (oo-choh)	9 **nueve** (noo-weh-veh)	10 **diez** (dee-yes?)

This is normal.

Esto es normal.
(S-toh s nohr-mal.)

You are doing well.

Usted está muy bien.
(Oo-steth s-ta moo-ee bee-n.)

Push!

¡Empuje!
(M-poo-heh!)

Don't push!

¡No empuje!
(Noh m-poo-heh!)

Breathe!	**¡Respire!** *(Res-peer-ay!)*
You need a Caesarian section.	**Usted necesita una sección cesareana.** *(Oo-steth ness-e-see-ta oo-na seck-see-ohn seh-sar-ee-an-a.)*
Congratulations!	**¡Felicitaciones!** *(Fell-ees-ee-tas-ee-ohn-ehs!)*
It's a boy!	**¡Es un muchacho!** *(S un moo-cha-choh!)*
It's a girl!	**¡Es una muchacha!** *(S una-moo-cha-cha!)*
The baby needs special care.	**El bebé necesita cuidado especial.** *(L beh-beh ness-eh-see-ta kwee-da-thoh s-pes-ee-al.)*

Chapter 9

Neurological

Cultural Notes: As the Latino population has a high incidence of hypertension and cardiovascular disease, the risk for cerebrovascular disorders is increased.

The high incidence of diabetes in this population increases the risk for neuropathies and diabetic retinopathy.

Helpful Hints:

- Monitor neurologic status for strokes.
- Monitor for parasthesias and visual disorders.

Do you have a headache?	¿Tiene Usted dolor de cabeza? (Tee-en-eh oo-steth doh-lohr deh ka-beh-sa?)
Do you have frequent headaches?	¿Tiene dolores de cabeza frecuentes? (Tee-en-eh doh-lohr-ehs deh ka-beh-sa free-ku-when-tehs?)
Do you have numbness or tingling anywhere?	¿Tiene adormecido o sensación de hormigueo en alguna parte? (Tee-en-eh ah-dor-meh-see-thoh oh sen-sa-see-ohn deh or-mee-geh-oh n al-goon-a par-teh?)
Point to it.	Señálelo. (Sen-ya-leh-loh.)
Can you feel this?	¿Siente esto? (See-n-teh s-toh?)

Neurological	Neurological
(Check for pain or sensation)	
Did you lose consciousness?	**¿Perdió el conocimiento?** *(Pehr-dee-oh L kohn-oh-seem-ee-n-toh?)*
Do you lose your balance?	**¿Perdió el equilibrio?** *(Pehr-dee-oh L ehk-ee-leeb-ree-oh?)*
Do you have seizures?	**¿Tiene ataques?** *(Tee-en-eh ah-tah-kehs?)*
Do you have tremors?	**¿Tiene sensación de temblor?** *(Tee-en-eh sen-sa-see-ohn deh tem-blohr?)*
Is your neck stiff?	**¿Está su cuello rígido?** *(S-ta soo kweh-yoh ree-hee-thoh?)*
Does your neck hurt?	**¿Le duele el cuello?** *(Leh doo-well-eh L kwell-yo?)*
Does the light hurt your eyes?	**¿Le duelen los ojos con la luz?** *(Leh dew-well-n lohs oh-hohs kohn la loose?)*

Do you have trouble remembering things?	**¿Tiene problemas para recordar cosas?**
	(Tee-en-eh proh-blehme-as pa-ra reh-kord-are ko-sas?)
Do you see flashing lights?	**¿Ve luces como destellos?**
	(Veh loos-ehs koh-moh dehs-teh-yohs?)
Do you see floating objects?	**¿Ve objetos que flotan?**
	(Veh ob-het-ohs k flo-tan?)
Do you have blurred vision?	**¿Tiene la visión borrosa?**
	(Tee-en-eh la v-see-ohn boh-roh-sa?)

Chapter 10

Musculoskeletal

Cultural Notes: Obesity, common in the Hispanic population, may lead to joint problems in the hips and knees. A high incidence of diabetes increases the risk for foot problems.

Helpful Hints:

- Assess for joint pain in knees and hips
- Assess feet for circulation, ulcers, and paresthesias.

Can you walk?	**¿Puede Usted caminar?** *(Pu-weh-theh oo-steth kah-men-ar?)*
Do you need help walking?	**¿Necesita Usted ayuda para caminar?** *(Nes-eh-see-ta oo-steth a-yo-tha pa-ra ka-men-ar?)*
Do you use a wheelchair?	**¿Usa Usted una silla de ruedas?** *(Oo-sa oo-steth oo-na see-ya deh roo-way-thas?)*
crutches?	**¿Usa Usted muletas?** *(Oo-sa oo-steth moo-let-as?)*
a cane?	**¿Usa Usted un bastón?** *(Oo-sa oo-steth oon bas-thohn?)*
Can you move your hands?	**¿Puede Usted mover las manos?** *(Pu-weh-theh oo-steth mo-vehr las ma-nohs?)*
fingers?	**¿los dedos?** *(los-deh-thohs?)*

Musculoskeletal

Musculoskeletal	Musculoskeletal
arms?	**¿los brazos?**
	(los bra-sohs)
legs?	**¿las piernas?**
	(las pee-ehr-nas?)
toes?	**¿los dedos del pie?**
	(los deh-thohs del-pee-eh?)
Can you feel this?	**¿Puede Usted sentir esto?**
	(Poo-weh-they oo-steth sen-teer s-toh?)
Do you have pain? (See Chapter 1)	**¿Tiene Usted dolor?**
(Check for pain or sensation.)	*(Tee-en-neh oo-steth doh-lohr?)*

Chapter 11

Psychiatric Conditions

Cultural Notes: As with most cultures, Latinos are hesitant to admit to psychiatric disorders. There may be a higher incidence of post-traumatic stress disorder and acute paranoid reactions which may lead to social isolation. In keeping with their external locus of control, Latinos may feel external forces as being responsible for their psychiatric problems. They may not present to the health care provider at all, instead using family for support with their problems.

Latinos also are not unlike other cultures in that they use alcohol as a way of celebrating life, but alcoholism is a crucial health problem for Mexican Americans.

Puerto Ricans are known to experience **susto,** a sudden fright caused by shock. They are also susceptible to an **ataque,** where they fall to the ground, screaming and moving their legs and arms uncontrollably.

Helpful Hints:

- If it is felt that the individual is at risk, an interpreter should be summoned to assist in a psychiatric evaluation.

- Apply helpful hints suggested in Chapter 12, "Emergency Room Visits," related to emotionalism typical in this culture.

- Be sensitive to questions related to alcoholic intake.

- Enlist the assistance of family members with outbursts. Allow the client to express emotions that are culturally appropriate. Consider the need for further evaluation.

Do you want to hurt yourself?	**¿Quiere Usted lastimarse?** (*Kee-ehr-a oo steth la-steem-ar-seh?*)
Do you want to hurt someone else?	**¿Quiere Usted lastimar a otra persona?** (*Kee-ehr-eh oo-steth la-steem-ar ah oh-tra pehr-sohn-ah?*)
Did you lose your job?	**¿Perdió Usted su trabajo?** (*Pehr-dee-oh oo-steth soo tra-ba-ho?*)
Did you lose a family member?	**¿Perdió Usted a un miembro de su familia?** (*Pehr-dee-oh oo-steth oon me-eem-broh deh soo fa-meel-ee-ah?*)
Did you lose a friend?	**¿Perdió Usted a un/una amigo/a?** (*Pehr-dee-oh oo-steth ooneh/o ona ah-mee-goh/gah?*)
Do you feel out of control?	**¿Se siente Usted fuera de control?** (*Seh see-en-teh oo-steth foo-ehr-ah deh kohn-trohl?*)

Psychiatric Conditions	Psychiatric Conditions
Do you hear voices?	¿Oye Usted voces? *(Oh-yeh oo-steth voh-sehs?)*
Do you sleep at night?	¿Durmió Usted en la noche? *(Dur-me-oh oo-steth ehn-lah-noh-cheh?)*
Are you under a lot of stress?	¿Tiene mucho estrés? *(Tee-en-eh oo-steth moo-choh eh-strehs?)*
Are you depressed?	¿Está Usted deprimido/a? *(S-ta oo-steth deh-pree-meh-thoh/thah?)*
Are you anxious?	¿Está Usted ansioso/a? *(S-ta oo-steth ahn-see-oh-soh/sah?)*
Are you nervous?	¿Está Usted nervioso/a? *(S-ta oo-steth nehr-v-oh-soh/sah?)*
Are you angry?	¿Está Usted enojado/a? *(S-ta oo-steth n-oh-hah-thoh/tha?)*
Do you drink alcohol?	¿Bebe Usted alcohol? *(Beh-beh oo-steth al-koh-hah!?)*
Beer?	¿Cerveza? *(Sehr-vehs-sa?)*

Whiskey?	**¿Whiskey?** *(Wees-kee?)*
Vodka?	**¿Vodka?** *(Vohd-ka?)*
Wine?	**¿Vino?** *(Vee-no?)*
Gin?	**¿Ginebra?** *(Gee-neh-bra?)*
How much?	**¿Cuánto?** *(Kwan-toh)*
How many bottles a day?	**¿Cuántas botellas al día?** *(Kwan-tahs boh-teh-yas al dee-ah?)*
How many glasses a day?	**¿Cuántos vasos al día?** *(Kwan-toh vah-sohs al dee-ah?)*

Chapter 12

Emergency Room Visits

Cultural Notes: People of Latino origin, including those coming from or who have family origins in southern Europe, may tend to become more emotional than individuals from other parts of the world. Clients of Latino or Spanish-speaking descent may appear to react to medical conditions, especially emergencies, in an extraordinarily dramatic manner. These may include verbal threats, gestures of suicide, pseudoseizures, fainting, shouting, or other similar reactions. **Susto** and **ataque** are examples of folk diseases that may be seen. **Susto** is a "shock" caused by a sudden fright. **Ataque** is where the person falls to the ground, screaming and moving legs and arms uncontrollably. These behaviors may not always indicate any pathology when considered within a broad cultural perspective, but may require psychiatric evaluation.

This population has strong family ties and may arrive in the emergency room with many family members. The male is considered the chief decision maker, but decisions are made within the family context.

It is important to remember that children may be called upon to interpret for parents.

In case of injury caused by domestic violence, Latino patients may be reluctant to assess the blame for their injuries. Many medications that require a prescription in the United States may be purchased over the counter in Latin America.

Helpful Hints:

- Ask your client to relax as much as possible. Reassure him/her that procedures and operations that may appear to be dramatic are often routine in today's world.

- Acknowledge the client's emotionalism by speaking in a calm voice, offering words of assurance and confidence about the care he/she is receiving.

- Do not interrupt clients when they are expressing their concerns. Let them know that you are taking their concerns seriously.

- Acknowledge the decision maker in the individual family, but include the entire family in the decisions.
- Consider the appropriateness of children as interpreters, especially with limited medical terminology and the topic at hand.
- Explain to Latino clients that although some family matters may appear to be private in some other cultures, in the United States injuries should be reported to the police. Criminal investigation and charges may be filed.
- Anticipate large numbers of family and relatives. Provide space and acceptance for family cultural values.
- Carefully assess all medications being taken.

Introductions/Instructions

Can I help you?

¿En qué le puedo servir?
(Ehn keh-poo-eh-thoh seer-veer-leh?)

Do you speak English?

¿Habla Usted inglés?
(Ah-bla oo-steth een-gl-ehs?)

I do not speak Spanish.

No hablo español.
(No ah-bloh s-pahn-yoh-l.)

What is your name?

¿Cómo se llama Usted?
(Koh-moh seh yah-mah oo-steth?)

Do you need a wheelchair?

¿Necesita una silla de ruedas?
(Ness-eh-see-tah oon-ah see-ya deh roo-way-thahs?)

Is there someone we should call?

¿Hay alguien que debemos llamar?
(Eye al-geeyen k deh-beh-mohs yah-mar?)

Emergency Room Visits

Write the name and telephone number here.

Escriba el nombre y el número de teléfono aquí.
(S-kree-bah l nowm-breh deh L noo-meh-roh deh tel-eh-fan-oh ah-key?)

Lie on the stretcher.

Acuéstese en la camilla.
(Ah-koo-west-eh-seh n la kam-ee-ya.)

The doctor is coming soon.

El doctor viene pronto.
(L doc-tor vee-ehn-eh prohn-toh.)

Take off your shirt/blouse.

Quítese la camisa/la blusa.
(Kee-tehs-seh la ka-mee-sa/la bloo-sa.)

Take off your clothes.

Quítese la ropa.
(Kee-teh-seh la roh-pa.)

Put on this johnny.

Póngase la bata.
(Pon-ga-seh la ba-ta.)

Take off your shoes.

Quítese los zapatos.
(Kee-teh-seh lohs sa-pat-tohs.)

Assessment

(Refer to separate body systems for other assessments.)

I need to examine you.	**Tengo que examinarlo/la.** *(Ten-go k x-a-mean-are-lo/la.)*
How old are you?	**¿Cuántos años tiene Usted?** *(Kwan-tohs ahn-yohs tee-en-eh oo-steth?)*
Do you have	Tiene Usted *(Tee-en-eh oo-steth)*
high blood pressure?	**¿la presión alta?** *(La pres-ee-ohn al-ta?)*
heart problems?	**¿problemas del corazón?** *(pro-blehm-as del coihr-a-sohn?)*
a pacemaker?	**¿un marcapasos?** *(oon mar-ka-pa-sohs?)*

Emergency Room Visits	Emergency Room Visits
diabetes?	¿diabetes? *(dee-a-bay-tace?)*
kidney failure?	¿insuficiencia renal? *(in-suf-is-e-en-see-a ree-nah!?)*
hepatitis?	¿hepatitis? *(hep-a-tee-teas?)*
cancer?	¿cáncer? *(kan-sir?)*
Where is the cancer?	¿Dónde está el cáncer? *(Dohn-deh s-ta L kan-sehr)*
Do you have glaucoma?	¿Tiene Usted glaucoma? *(Tee-en-eh oo-steth glau-kohm-ah?)*
cataracts?	¿cataratas? *(kat-ah-rah-tas?)*
diverticulitis?	¿diverticulitis? *(dee-vehr-teeck-yoo-lee-tees?)*
Crohn's disease	¿la enfermedad de Crohn? *(la n-fehr-meh-dath deh Crohn.)*

colitis?	**¿colitis?** *(kol-ee-tees?)*
HIV/AIDS?	**¿Sida?** *(see- thah?)*
a sexually transmitted disease?	**¿una enfermedad transmitida sexualmente?** *(oo-na n-fehr-meh-dath trans-mee-tee- theh sex-oo-al-mehn-teh?)*
Do you take medicines?	**¿Toma Usted medicinas?** *(Toh-ma oo-steth mehd-ee-seen-as?)*
Can you write them down?	**¿Puede escribirlas?** *(Poo-weh-theh s-kree-beer-las?)*
Did you take any poisons?	**¿Tomó Usted veneno?** *(To-moh oo-steth vehn-eh-noh?)*
Can you write them down?	**¿Puede escribirlas?** *(poo-weh-theh s-kree-beer-las?)*

Emergency Room Visits **57**

Pain Assessment (See Chapter 1)	
Do you have a fever?	**¿Tiene Usted fiebre (calentura)?** *(Tee-en-eh oo-steth fee-ehb-reh/kal-en-too-ra?)*
Are you pregnant?	**¿Está Usted embarazada?** *(S-ta oo-steth m-bar-ah-sa-tha?)*
When is your baby due?	**¿Cuándo nace su bebé?** *(k-wan-doh na-seh soo beh-beh?)*
Diagnostic Tests	
You need an EKG.	**Usted necesita un electrocardiograma.** *(Oo-steth ness-eh-see-ta oon eh-lec-troh-car-dee-oh-gram-ah.)*
X-Ray.	**un examen de rayos X.** *(Oon x-ah-men deh ray-ohs eck-ease.)*
MRI.	**Un examen de imagen de resonancia magnética.** *(Oon-x-ah-men deh ee-mah-hen deh rehs-ohn-ahn-see-ah mag-neh-tee-kah.)*

PET Scan.	**un escaneo PET.** *(oon-can-eh-oh PehEhTeh.)*
cast.	**un yeso.** *(oon yes-oh.)*
operation.	**una operación, cirugía.** *(oo-nah oh-pehr-ah-see-ohn, seer-oo-hee-ah.)*
intravenous	**intravenosa.** *(een-tra-vehn-ehn-oh-sa.)*
medication.	**medicina.** *(mehd-ee-see-na.)*
stitches.	**puntadas.** *(poon-tah-thas.)*
You have a broken bone.	**Usted tiene un hueso roto.** *(oo-steth tee-en-eh oon weh-soh roh-toh.)*
sprain.	**torcedura.** *(tor-seh-door-a.)*

Emergency Room Visits	Emergency Room Visits
collapsed lung.	**colapso del pulmón.** *(ko-lap-soh del pool-mohn.)*
concussion.	**concusión.** *(kon-coos-eh-ohn.)*
contusion.	**contusión.** *(kohn-too-see-ohn.)*
infection.	**infección.** *(een-fehk-see-ohn.)*
bladder infection.	**infección de la vejiga.** *(een-fehk-see-ohn deh la veh-hee-ga.)*
kidney infection.	**infección de los riñones.** *(een-fehk-see-ohn day lohs reen-yohn-ehs.)*
heart attack.	**ataque al corazón.** *(ah-ta-keh al kohr-ah-sohn.)*
stroke.	**infarto.** *(een-far-toh.)*

Appendix A

Common Conversation

Cultural Notes: Latinos typically do not disclose personal information or trust others until they have established a relationship. It is best to engage in small talk initially and to address individuals by formal names until they are comfortable.

Helpful Hints:

- Address clients formally until you have become acquainted with them.
- Engage in small talk before starting the assessment to establish a relationship and trust.
- Reserve any kidding or teasing (initially considered rude) until a relationship has been established.

Common Conversation

Common Conversation	
Good morning.	**Buenos días.** (Boo-weh-nohs dee-ahs.)
Good afternoon.	**Buenas tardes.** (Boo-wey-nahs tar-dehs.)
Good night.	**Buenas noches.** (Boo-weh-nahs noh-chehs.)
Excuse me.	**Perdóneme.** (Pehr-d-ohn-ah-meh.)
I'm sorry.	**Lo siento.** (Loh see-n-toh.)
Please.	**Por Favor.** (Pohr fah-vohr.)
Thank you.	**Gracias.** (grah-see-ahs.)
Yes.	**Sí** (See.)

No.	**No** *(Noh.)*
Maybe.	**Tal vez** *(Tal vehs.)*
I don't know.	**No sé.** *(Noh seh.)*
May I come in?	**¿Puedo pasar?** *(Poo-weh-thoh pa-sare?)*
Very good.	**Muy bien.** *(Moo-ee bee-n.)*
My name is _____.	**Me llamo_____.** *(Meh yahm-oh _____.)*
I am your nurse.	**Soy su enfermero/a.** *(Soy soo n-fehr-mehr-oh/ah.)*
Nice to meet you.	**Es un gusto conocerlo/la.** *(S oon goo-stoh koh-noh-sehr-lo/la.)*

Common Conversation

Common Conversation	
Do you speak English?	**¿Habla Usted inglés?** *(Ah-bla oo-steth een-glehs.)*
I do not speak Spanish.	**No hablo español.** *(No a-bloh s-pan-yo-hl.)*
I do not understand.	**No comprendo.** *(No com-pren-doh.)*
Very good.	**Muy bien.** *(Moo-ee bee-n.)*
Instructions/Care	
I need to examine you.	**Tengo que examinarlo/la.** *(Tehn-goh k x-ah-meen-ar-lo/la.)*
The doctor is coming soon.	**El doctor viene pronto.** *(L dohc-tohr vee-ehn-eh prohn-toh.)*
Take off your shirt/blouse.	**Quítese la camisa/la blusa.** *(Kee-teh-seh la ka-mees-sa/la bloo-sa.)*

Take off your clothes.	**Quítese la ropa.** *(Kee-teh-sey la roh-pa.)*
Put on this johnny.	**Póngase la bata.** *(Pon-ga-seh la ba-ta.)*
Take off your shoes.	**Quítese los zapatos.** *(Kee-teh-seh lohs sa-pat-ohs.)*
Lie down.	**Acuéstese.** *(A-koo-west-eh-say.)*
Sit up.	**Póngase derecho.** *(Pohn-ga-seh deh-reh-ch-oh.)*
Sit down.	**Siéntese.** *(See-en-teh-seh.)*
Stand up.	**Póngase de pie.** *(Pohn-ga-seh deh pee-eh.)*
Open your mouth.	**Abra la boca.** *(A-bra la boh-ka.)*

Common Conversation	Common Conversation
You must stay in bed.	**Tiene que quedarse en la cama.** *(Tee-en-eh k keh-dar-seh n la ka-ma.)*
I have some medicine for you.	**Tengo medicina para Usted.** *(Ten-goh mehd-eh-seen-ah pa-ra-oo-steth.)*
I have to give you an injection (shot.)	**Tengo que darle una inyección.** *(Ten-go k dar-leh oo-na in-yek-see-ohn.)*
I am going to take your blood pressure.	**Voy a tomar la presión de la sangre.** *(Voy ah toh-mare la press-eh-ohn deh la san-greh.)*
I am going to take your temperature.	**Voy a tomar su temperatura.** *(Voy ah toh-mar soo tem-pehr-ah-tour-ah.)*
We need a urine sample.	**Necesitamos una muestra de la orina.** *(Ness-eh-see-ta-mhos oo-na moo-ehs-tra deh la oh-reen-ah.)*
blood sample.	**de la sangre.** *(deh la sahn-greh.)*

stool sample.	del excremento. (del x-kreh-mehn-toh.)
sputum sample.	del esputo. (del s-poo-toh.)
This will hurt a little bit/a lot.	Esto va a doler un poco/mucho. (S-toh va ah doh-lohr oon poh-koh/moo-choh.)
Are you hungry?	¿Tiene Usted hambre? (Tee-en-eh oo-steth ham-breh?)
Are you thirsty?	¿Tiene Usted sed? (Tee-en-eh oo-steth seth?)
Are you cold?	¿Tiene frío? (Tee-en-eh free-oh?)
Are you hot?	¿Tiene calor? (Tee-en-eh ka-lor?)
Did you sleep well last night?	¿Durmió bien anoche? (Door-mee-oh bee-n ah-noh-cheh?)

Common Conversation	Common Conversation
Was there noise?	**¿Hubo ruido?** *(Oo-boh roo-ee-thoh?)*
Were you in pain?	**¿Sintió dolor?** *(Seen-tee-oh doh-lohr?)*
When did you move your bowels last?	**¿Cuándo fue la última vez que tuvo una evacuación?** *(Kwan-doh foo-weh la ool-tee-ma vehs k too-voh oo-na eh-vak-oo-ahs-ee-own?)*
Do you need a laxative?	**¿Necesita un laxante?** *(Ness-eh-see-ta oo-na lax-ahn-teh?)*
I need to weigh you.	**Tengo que pesarlo/la.** *(Ten-goh k peh-sahr-lo/la.)*
Please step on the scale.	**Póngase en la báscula, por favor.** *(Pon-ga-seh n la bas-koo-la poh-la poh-r-fah-vohr.)*
It's time for your bath.	**Ya es la hora para su baño.** *(Ya s la oh-ra pa-ra soo bah-nyoh.)*

Here is some soap and water.

Aquí tiene jabón y agua.
(Ah-key tee-n-eh ha-bohn e eh-gwa.)

a towel.

Una toalla.
(Oo-na toh-ay-ya.)

a facecloth.

Una toallita.
(Oo-na toh-ay-ee-ta.)

Would you like to shave?

¿Quiere afeitarse?
(Key-ehr-eh ah-fay-tar-say?)

Would you like to take a shower?

¿Quiere tomar una ducha?
(Kee-ehr-eh toh-mar oo-na doo-cha?)

The Room

Push this button to call the nurse.

Empuje este botón para llamar al/a la/enfermero/a.
(M-poo-heh s-teh boh-tohn pa-ra ya-mar ahl-la n-fehr-mehr-ah.)

Common Conversation

Common Conversation	
Use this button to turn on the television.	**Use este botón para poner la televisión.** *(Oo-séh s-teh boh-tohn pa-ra po-nehr la tel-eh-vees-ee-ohn.)*
Do you need a blanket?	**¿Necesita una cobija?** *(Ness-eh-see-ta oo-na ko-bee-ha?)*
Do you want another pillow?	**¿Quiere otra almohada?** *(Kee-ehr-eh oh-tra al-moh-ah-tha?)*
Dial _____ to get an outside telephone line.	**Marque _____ para una línea fuera del hospital.** *(Mar-keh _____ pa-ra oo-na lee-n-eh-ah foo-ehr-a del oh-spee-tal.)*

Appendix B

Colors-Time-Numbers

Colors	Colores
black	**negro** *(neh-groh)*
blue	**azul** *(ah-sool)*
brown	**castaño, café** *(cas-tan-yo/ca-feh)*
green	**verde** *(vehr-deh)*
orange	**anaranjado** *(ah-nar-an-hado)*
pink	**rosado** *(roh-sa-thoh)*
purple	**púrpura, morado** *(poor-poor-ah, mohr-a-thoh)*
red	**rojo** *(roh-hoh)*

English	Spanish	Pronunciation
white	**blanco**	(blan-koh)
yellow	**amarillo**	(ah-mar-eel-yoh)
dark	**oscuro**	(oh-skoor-oh)
light	**claro**	(klahr-oh)
Time	**tiempo**	(tee-em-poh)
hour	**hora**	(or-ah)
minutes	**minutos**	(me-noo-tohs)
morning	**mañana**	(man-yan-ah)

noon	**mediodia** *(meh-dee-oh-dee-ah)*
afternoon	**tarde** *(tar-deh)*
night	**noche** *(no-cheh)*
day	**dia** *(dee-ah)*
week	**semana** *(seh-man-ah)*
month	**mes** *(mehs)*
year	**año** *(an-yo)*
Days of the week	**Días de la Semana** *(Dee-ahs deh la seh-man-ah)*

Monday	**lunes** *(loo-nehs)*
Tuesday	**martes** *(mar-tehs)*
Wednesday	**miércoles** *(mee-ehr-ko-lehs)*
Thursday	**jueves** *(who-eh-vehs)*
Friday	**viernes** *(vee-ehr-nehs)*
Saturday	**sábado** *(sa-ba-thoh)*
Sunday	**domingo** *(doh-meen-goh)*
Week	**semana** *(seh-man-ah)*
Months of the year	**Meses del año** *(meh-ses del an-yoh)*

Colors-Time-Numbers	Colors-Time-Numbers
January	**enero** *(en-ehr-oh)*
February	**febrero** *(feb-rehr-oh)*
March	**marzo** *(mar-soh)*
April	**abril** *(ah-bril)*
May	**mayo** *(my-oh)*
June	**junio** *(hoon-ee-oh)*
July	**julio** *(jool-ee-oh)*
August	**agosto** *(ah-go-stow)*
September	**septiembre** *(sep-tee-em-breh)*

October	**octubre**
	(ohk-too-breh)
November	**noviembre**
	(no-vehm-breh)
December	**diciembre**
	(dee-see-em-breh)
Seasons	**Estaciones**
Fall	**otoño**
	(oh-tohn-yo)
Winter	**invierno**
	(in-vee-air-no)
Spring	**primavera**
	(pree-mah-vehr-ah)
Summer	**verano**
	(vair-ah-noh)
Numbers	**Números**
	(noo-mer-ohs)

Colors-Time-Numbers

1	2	3	4	5
uno *oo-noh*	**dos** *(dohs)*	**tres** *(trehs)*	**cuatro** *(kwa-tro)*	**cinco** *(sin-ko)*
6	7	8	9	10
seis *(sais)*	**siete** *(see-et-teh)*	**ocho** *(oh-choh)*	**nueve** *(new-eh-veh)*	**diez** *(dee-es)*
11	12	13	14	15
once *(ohn-seh)*	**doce** *(doh-seh)*	**trece** *(treh-seh)*	**catorce** *(ka-tor-seh)*	**quince** *(keen seh)*
16	17	18	19	20
diez y seis *(dee-es e sais)*	**diez y siete** *(dee-es e see-et-teh)*	**diez y ocho** *(dee-es e oh-choh)*	**diez y nueve** *(dee-es e noo-eh-veh)*	**veinte** *(vain-teh)*
21	22	23	24	25
veinte y uno	**veinte y dos**	**veinte y tres**	**veinte y cuatro**	**veinte y cinco**

26 veinte y seis	27 veinte y siete	28 veinte y ocho	29 veinte y nueve	30 treinta (tray-ain-ta)
31 treinta y uno	32 treinta y dos	33 treinta y tres	34 treinta y cuatro	35 treinta y cinco
36 treinta y seis	37 treinta y siete	38 treinta y ocho	39 treinta y nueve	40 curaenta (kwar-en-ta)
41 cuarenta y uno	42 cuarenta y dos	43 cuarenta y tres	44 cuarenta y cuatro	45 cuarenta y cinco
46 cuarenta y seis	47 cuarenta y siete	48 cuarenta y ocho	49 cuarenta y nueve	50 cincuenta (sin-kwen-ta)
51 cincuenta y uno	52 cincuenta y dos	53 cincuenta y tres	54 cincuenta y cuatro	55 cincuenta y cinco

Colors-Time-Numbers

56 cincuenta y seis	57 cincuenta y siete	58 cincuenta y ocho	59 cincuenta y nueve	60 sesenta (ses-en-ta)
61 sesenta y uno	62 sesenta y dos	63 sesenta y tres	64 sesenta y cuatro	65 sesenta y cinco
66 sesenta y seis	67 sesenta y siete	68 sesenta y ocho	69 sesenta y nueve	70 setenta (set-ten-ta)
71 setenta y uno	72 setenta y dos	73 setenta y tres	74 setenta y cuatro	75 setenta y cinco
76 setenta y seis	77 setenta y siete	78 setenta y ocho	79 setenta y nueve	80 ochenta (oh-chen-ta)

81 ochenta y uno	82 ochenta y dos	83 ochenta y tres	84 ochenta y cuatro	85 ochenta y cinco
86	87	88	89	90
ochenta y seis	ochenta y siete	ochenta y ocho	ochenta y nueve	noventa (no-ven-ta)
91	92	93	94	95
noventa y uno	noventa y dos	noventa y tres	noventa y cuatro	noventa y cinco
96	97	98	99	100
noventa y seis	noventa y siete	noventa y ocho	noventa y nueve	cien (see-en)

Appendix C

Vocabulary

apple	**manzana** (man-zan-ah)
arm	**brazo** (bra-soh)
abdomen	**abdomen** (ab-doh-men)
ankle	**tobillo** (toh-bee-yoh)
armpit	**axila/sobaco** (ax-eel-ah/soh-ba-koh)
back	**espalda** (s-pal-da)
banana	**plátano** (pla-ta-noh)
bathroom	**baño** (ban-yoh)

Vocabulary	Vocabulary
beans	**frijoles** *(free-hohl-ehs)*
bed	**cama** *(ka-ma)*
beef	**bif** *(beef)*
bone	**hueso** *(weh-soh)*
blanket	**cobija** *(ko-bee-ha)*
blood	**sangre** *(san-greh)*
blood pressure cuff	**banda de tomar la presión** *(ban-da deh toh-mar la pres-see-ohn)*
bread	**pan** *(pahn)*

English	Spanish	Pronunciation
breakfast	**desayuno**	*(des-ah-yoo-noh)*
breast	**pecho**	*(peh-choh)*
bruise	**moretón**	*(mohr-eh-tohn)*
buttock	**nalga**	*(nal-ga)*
cake	**pastel**	*(pa-stel)*
cane	**bastón**	*(bah-stohn)*
carrots	**zanahorias**	*(zan-a-hor-ee-as)*
cereal	**cereal**	*(seh-ray-al)*

Vocabulary

Vocabulary	
chair	**silla** (see-ya)
chapel	**capilla** (ka-pee-ya)
cheek	**mejilla** (may-he-ya)
chest	**pecho** (pey-choh)
chicken	**pollo** (po-yo)
coffee	**café** (ka-feh)
chocolate	**chocolate** (cho-ko-lah-teh)
cold	**frío** (free-oh)

English	Spanish	Pronunciation
corn	**maíz**	*(my-ees)*
delivery room	**sala de partos**	*(sa-la deh par-tohs)*
dentures	**dentaduras**	*(den-tah-dur-ahs)*
dialysis	**diálisis**	*(dee-ah-lee-sees)*
doctor	**doctor**	*(dok-tor)*
door	**puerta**	*(pu-ehr-ta)*
ear	**oído**	*(oh-ee-thoh)*
eggs	**huevos**	*(way-vohs)*

Vocabulary

Vocabulary	Vocabulary
elbow	**codo** *(ko-thoh)*
elevator	**elevador** *(l-eh-veh-dohr)*
emergency room	**sala de emergencia** *(sa-la deh em-er-hen-see-ah)*
exit	**salida** *(sal-ee-thah)*
eye	**ojos** *(oh-hos)*
face	**cara** *(ka-ra)*
finger	**dedo** *(deh-thoh)*
fish	**pescado** *(pes-kah-do)*

forehead	**frente** (fren-teh)
floor	**piso** (pee-soh)
foot	**pie** (pee-eh)
fruit	**fruta** (fru-ta)
gift shop	**tienda de regalos** (tee-en-da deh reh-gal-ohs)
grapefruit	**toronja** (tohr-ohn-ha)
hair	**pelo** (peh loh)
hallway	**pasillo** (pa-see-yo)

Vocabulary	Vocabulary
ham	**jamón** *(ha-mohn)*
hamburger	**hamburguesa** *(am-bur-guess-sa)*
hand	**mano** *(mahn-o)*
head	**cabeza** *(ka-beh-sa)*
heel	**talón** *(ta-lohn)*
hospital	**hospital** *(oh-spee-tal)*
hot	**caliente** *(kal-ee-yen-teh)*

intensive care unit	**unidad de cuidado intensivo** *(oo-nee-dath deh kwee-da-thoh een-ten-see-va)*
intrevenous	**intravenosa** *(een-tra-vehn-oh-sa)*
juice	**jugo** *(who-go)*
knee	**rodilla** *(roh-dee-ya)*
leg	**pierna** *(pee-ehr-na)*
lemon	**limón** *(lee-moan)*
light	**luz** *(loose)*

Vocabulary	Vocabulary
lip	**labio** *(la-bee-oh)*
lunch	**comida** *(ko-mee-tha)*
main lobby	**entrada principal** *(en-tra-tha preen-see-pal)*
maternity ward	**unidad de maternidad** *(oo-nee-dath deh mat-er-nee-dath)*
meat	**carne** *(kar-neh)*
milk	**leche** *(leh-cheh)*
mouth	**boca** *(bo-ka)*

MRI	**imagen de resonancia magnética** *(ee-ma-hen deh res-oh-nan-see-ah mag-net-ee-ka)*
neck	**cuello** *(ku-well-yo)*
nerve	**nervio** *(ner-v-oh)*
nipple	**pezón** *(peh-sohn)*
nose	**nariz** *(nar-eece)*
nurse	**enfermera** *(en-fehr-mehr-ah)*
nursery	**cunero** *(ku-nehr-oh)*
operating room	**sala de operaciones** *(sa-la deh oh-pehr-ah-see-own-ehs)*

Vocabulary	Vocabulary
orange	**naranja** *(nar-an-hah)*
oxygen	**oxígeno** *(ohk-seehe-no)*
parking lot	**estacionamiento** *(es-tas-ee-ohn-ah-men-toh)*
pediatric ward	**unidad pediátrica** *(oo-nee-dath peh-dee-ah-tree-kah)*
penis	**pene** *(peh-neh)*
pillow	**almohada** *(al-moh-ah-tha)*
physical therapy	**terapia física** *(ter-a-pee-a fees-e-ka)*
potatoes	**papas** *(pa-pas)*

recovery room	**sala de recuperación** *(sa-la deh oh-pehr-ah-see-ohn)*
rectum	**recto** *(rec-toh)*
rice	**arroz** *(ah-rohs)*
room	**cuarto** *(kwar-toh)*
salad	**ensalada** *(en-sal-a-tha)*
sandwich	**sandwich** *(sahn-dweech)*
shoulder	**hombro** *(ohm-bro)*
siderail	**riel de los lados de la cama** *(ree-l deh los la-thoh deh la ka-ma)*

Vocabulary

Vocabulary	Vocabulary
skin	**piel** (pee-el)
soap	**jabón** (ha-bohn)
soft drink	**refresco** (reh-fres-ko)
soup	**sopa** (soh-pa)
squash	**calabaza** (kal-a-ba-sa)
stairs	**escaleras** (es-ka-lehr-s)
stitches	**puntadas** (poon-ta-thas)
stethoscope	**estetoscopio** (es-ter-s-koh-pee-oh)

stomach	**estómago** *(es-toh-ma-go)*
stretcher	**camilla** *(ka-me-ya)*
table	**mesa** *(may-sa)*
tea	**té** *(teh)*
teeth	**dientes** *(dee-n-tehs)*
television	**televisión** *(tel-e-vees-ee-ohn)*
thermometer	**termómetro** *(tehr-mo-me-troh)*
telephone	**teléfono** *(tel-eh-fo-no)*

Vocabulary	Vocabulary
throat	**garganta** (gar-gan-ta)
toast	**tostada** (toh-sta-tha)
toe	**dedo del pie** (deh-doh del-pee-eh)
tooth	**diente** (dee-n-teh)
towel	**toalla** (tow-al-ya)
vagina	**vagina** (va-hee-na)
vanilla	**vainilla** (va-ee-neel-ya)
waiting room	**sala de espera** (sa-la deh s-pehr-ah)

walker	**andadera**	(an-da-deh-rah)
washcloth	**toallita de la cara**	(toh-ah-ye-ta deh la ka-ra)
water	**agua**	(ah-gwa)
wheelchair	**silla de ruedas**	(see-ya deh pru-eh-thas)
window	**ventana**	(ven-tan-a)
wrist	**muñeca**	(mun-yeh-ka)
x-ray	**rayos x**	(reh-yohs eck-ees)
x-ray department	**departamento de rayos x**	(deh-par-ta-men-toh deh reh-ohs eck-ees)

Vocabulary

Selected Vocabulary Spanglish and Mexican-Border Spanish

Vocabulary	
x-ray machine	**máquina de rayos x**
	(ma-kee-na deh reh-ohs eck-ees)
blond	**güero/a**
	(gu-wear-o/a)
bus	**guagua**
	(gwa-gwa)
cake	**queque**
	(keh-keh)
child	**chamaco/a**
	(cha-mak-ko/ah)
child	**esquincle/a**
	(s-keen-seh/ah)
close friend, twin	**cuate**
	(ku-wat-eh)
coat	**coe**
	(ko-weh)

to freeze	**frisar** *(free-sar)*
furniture	**furnitura** *(fur-nee-toor-a)*
grocery store	**grocería** *(grow-sehr-ee-ah)*
hanging out (as at a particular place)	**hangeo** *(hang-eh-oh)*
hurry up/that's right	**ándele** *(an-da-leh)*
job	**chamba** *(cham-ba)*
Laundromat	**washetería** *(wash-eh-tehr-ee-a)*
to leak	**liqueo** *(lee-keh-oh)*
	OR
	liquear *(lee-keh-ar)*

Vocabulary	Vocabulary
lunch	**lonche** *(lohn-cheh)*
to have lunch	**lonchear** *(lohn-cheh-ar)*
money (slang)	**lana** *(la-na)*
nurse	**nursa** *(noor-sa)*
native or folk healer	**curandero/a** *(koor-an-dehr-oh/a)*
orange (in Puerto Rico)	**china** *(chee-na)*
policeman	**poli** *(po-lee)*
prescription	**prescripción** *(preh-screep-see-ohn)*
roof	**roofo** *(roof-oh)*

shaman or native healer	**chamán**	(sha-mahn)
short	**chaparro/a**	(chah-par-oh/ah)
ticket	**tickete**	(teek-eh-teh)
truck	**troca**	(tro-ka)
to type	**tipear**	(tee-peh-ar)
to work	**chambear**	(ch-am-beh-ar)
to wash	**washear**	(wash-eh-ar)
to work	**workear**	(work-eh-ar)
One who heals with herbs	**yerbero/a**	(yehr-behr-oh/ah)

Vocabulary	Vocabulary
I Saw (instead of standard form "vi")	**vide** *(vee-deh)*
What did you say?	**¿Mandé?** *(man-deh)*
Who cares?	**¿Ni modo?** *(Nee mo-thoh)*

Notes

_____

_____

_____

_____

_____

_____

_____

_____

_____

_____

_____

_____

_____

_____

_____

_____

_____

_____

_____

_____

_____

_____

_____

_____

_____

_____

_____

_____

_____

_____

_____

_____

_____

_____

_____

_____

_____

_____

_____

_____

_____

_____

_____

_____

_____

_____

_____

_____

_____

_____

ᵀA information can be obtained
ICGtesting.com
ʰe USA
³⁵161216
ᵛ⁄00016B/98/P

9 781449 647902